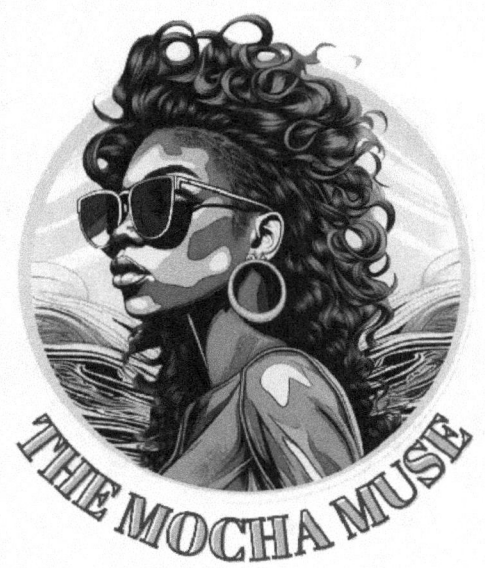

THE MOCHA MUSE

Thank you!

Thank You for Choosing "Just Keep Moving: Weight Loss Planner"!

Dear Reader,
We would like to express our heartfelt gratitude for your purchase of our book, "Just Keep Moving: Weight Loss Planner." as your companion on your weight loss journey. We are honored to be a part of your pursuit of a healthier, happier lifestyle.
To our readers, your trust in us means the world. We crafted "Just Keep Moving" with your needs in mind, aiming to provide a comprehensive resource that empowers you to make lasting lifestyle changes. Your commitment to self-improvement and dedication to your health is truly admirable.

Stay in touch!

DAY WILCOX
www.themochamuse.com

Empower Yourself with a Weight Loss Planner for Success

Getting in shape and losing weight requires a combination of healthy eating habits, regular physical activity, and a sustainable lifestyle. Here are some of the best ways to achieve your goals:

Set Realistic Goals: Start by setting achievable and realistic goals for yourself. Avoid aiming for drastic weight loss in a short period, as it can be unsustainable and unhealthy. Instead, focus on gradual and steady progress.

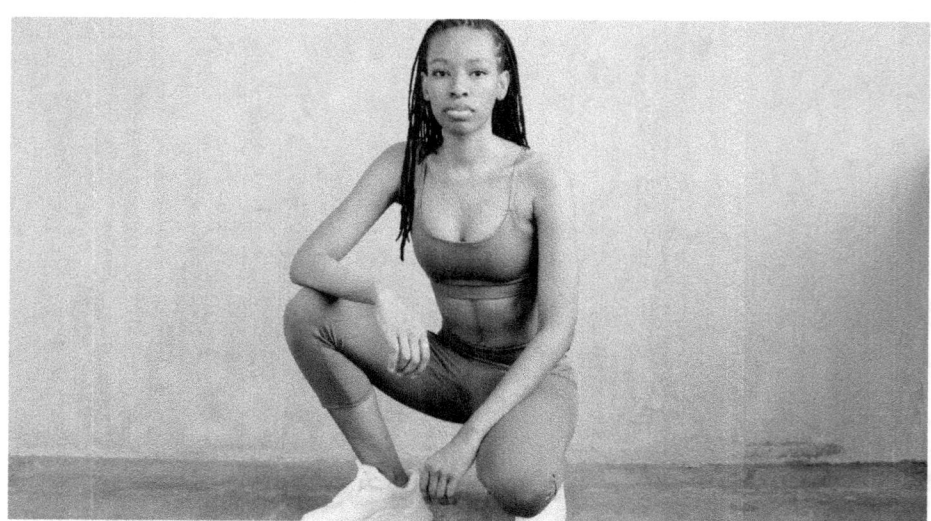

Transform Your Body and Mind

Balanced Diet: Adopt a balanced and nutritious diet. Include a variety of fruits, vegetables, whole grains, lean proteins, and healthy fats in your meals. Avoid or limit processed foods, sugary beverages, and excessive salt and sugar intake. Portion control is also important, so be mindful of your serving sizes.

Meal Planning: Plan your meals in advance to avoid impulsive and unhealthy food choices. Prepare your meals at home as much as possible, as it gives you better control over ingredients and portion sizes. Consider meal prepping for busy days to ensure you have healthy options readily available.

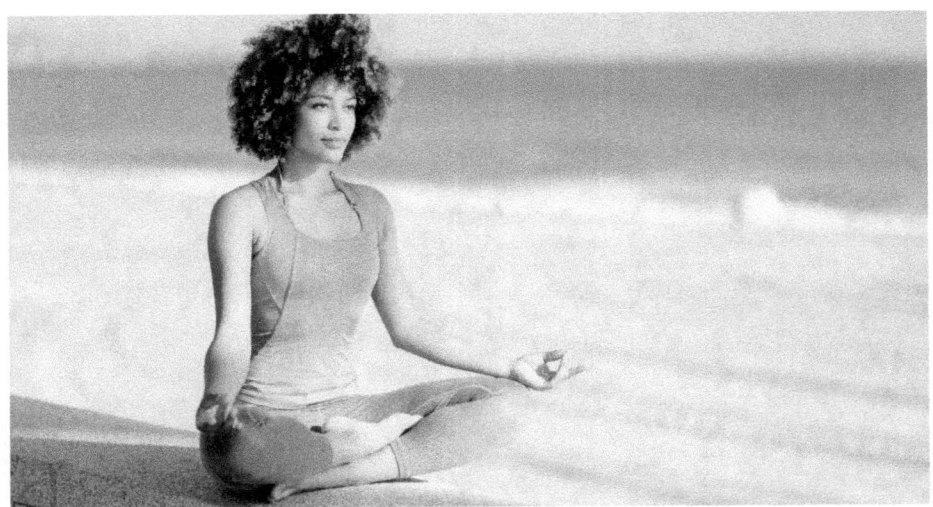

Stay Motivated and Reach Your Weight Loss Milestones

Regular Physical Activity: Engage in regular physical activity that suits your fitness level and preferences. Incorporate a mix of cardiovascular exercises (such as walking, running, cycling, or swimming) and strength training exercises (like weightlifting or bodyweight exercises) into your routine. Aim for at least 150 minutes of moderate-intensity aerobic activity or 75 minutes of vigorous-intensity activity per week, along with strength training exercises twice a week.

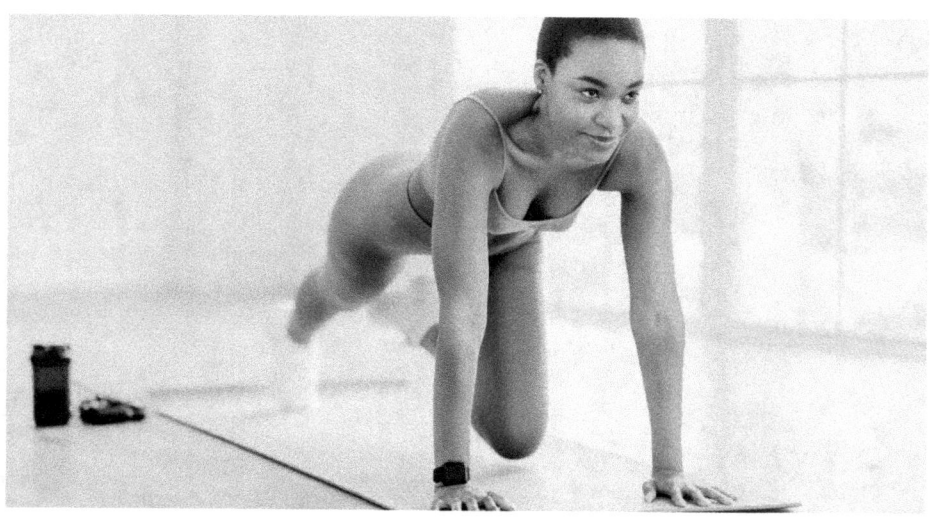

Your Personal Weight Loss Journey Companion

Find an Exercise Routine You Enjoy: Choose activities that you genuinely enjoy to make exercise a sustainable part of your lifestyle. It could be dancing, hiking, yoga, martial arts, or any other form of physical activity that keeps you engaged and motivated. Mix up your workouts to avoid boredom and keep challenging yourself.

Stay Consistent: Consistency is key when it comes to getting in shape and losing weight. Make exercise and healthy eating a regular part of your routine rather than occasional efforts. Even on days when you lack motivation, find ways to stay active and make mindful food choices.

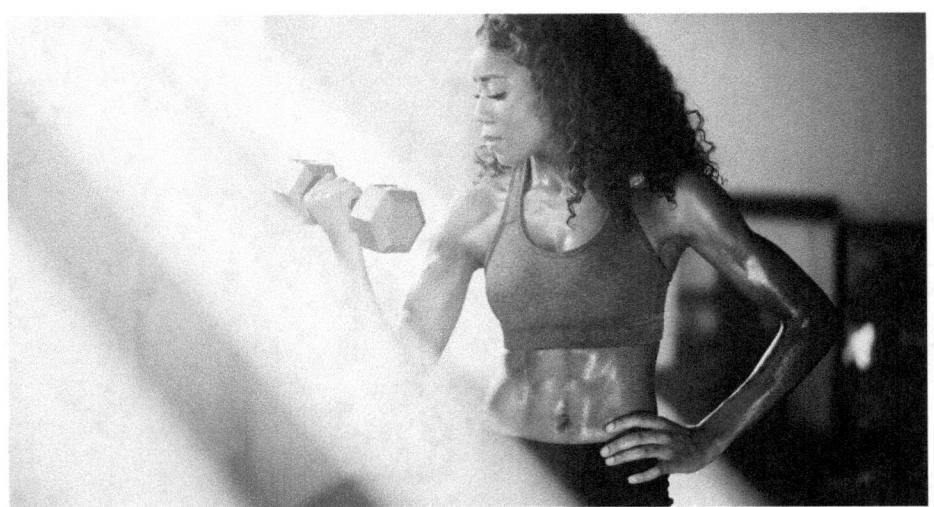

Achieving Weight Loss Goals

Stay Hydrated: Drink an adequate amount of water throughout the day. Water helps maintain hydration, supports metabolism, and can contribute to a feeling of fullness, which may help with portion control.

Get Sufficient Sleep: Prioritize quality sleep as it plays a vital role in weight management and overall well-being. Aim for 7-8 hours of sleep per night to allow your body to rest, recover, and regulate important hormones related to appetite and metabolism.

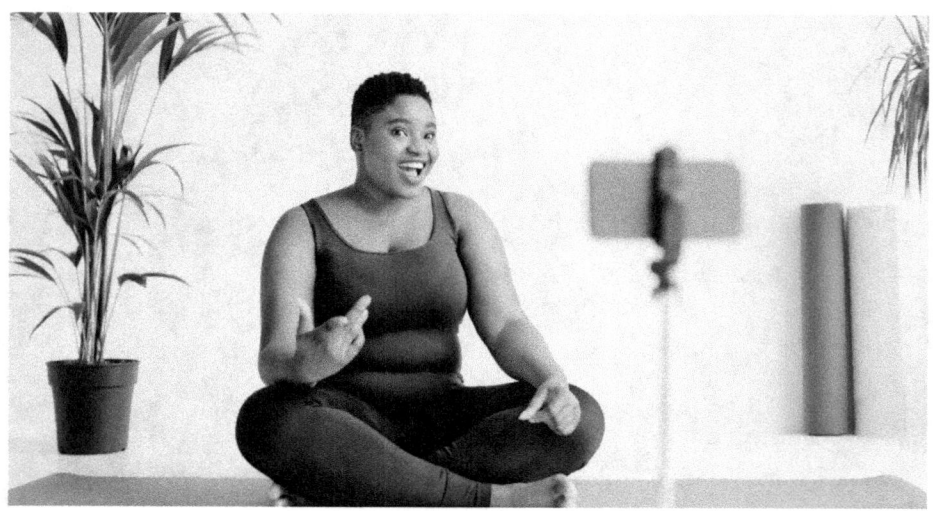

Your Roadmap to Sustainable Weight Loss

Manage Stress: Find healthy ways to manage stress, as it can impact your eating habits and overall health. Engage in activities like meditation, deep breathing exercises, journaling, or hobbies that help you relax and reduce stress levels.

Seek Support: Consider joining a support group, working with a personal trainer, or seeking guidance from a registered dietitian or nutritionist. Surrounding yourself with a supportive community can provide accountability, motivation, and valuable insights on your weight loss journey.

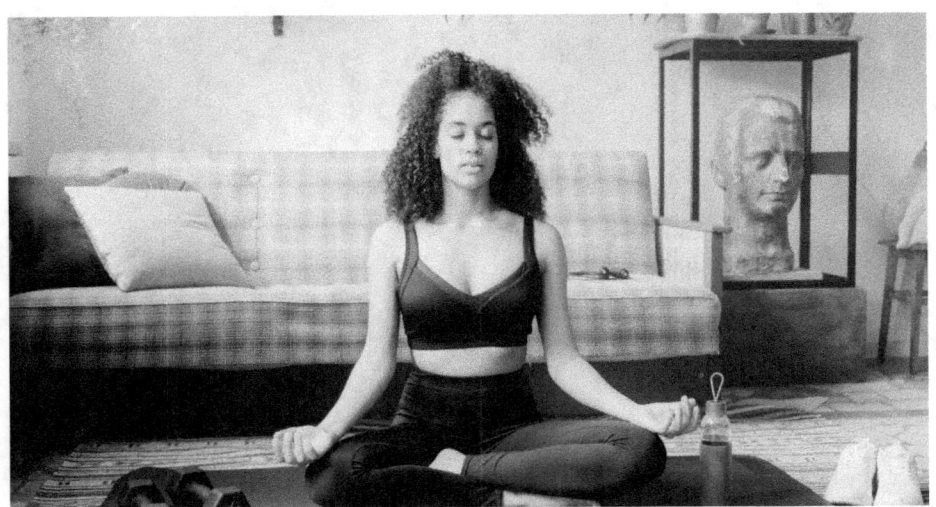

Unlock Your Potential with a Personalized Weight Loss

Remember, the key to sustainable weight loss is making long-term lifestyle changes rather than relying on quick fixes. Be patient, embrace a positive mindset, and celebrate each small victory along the way.

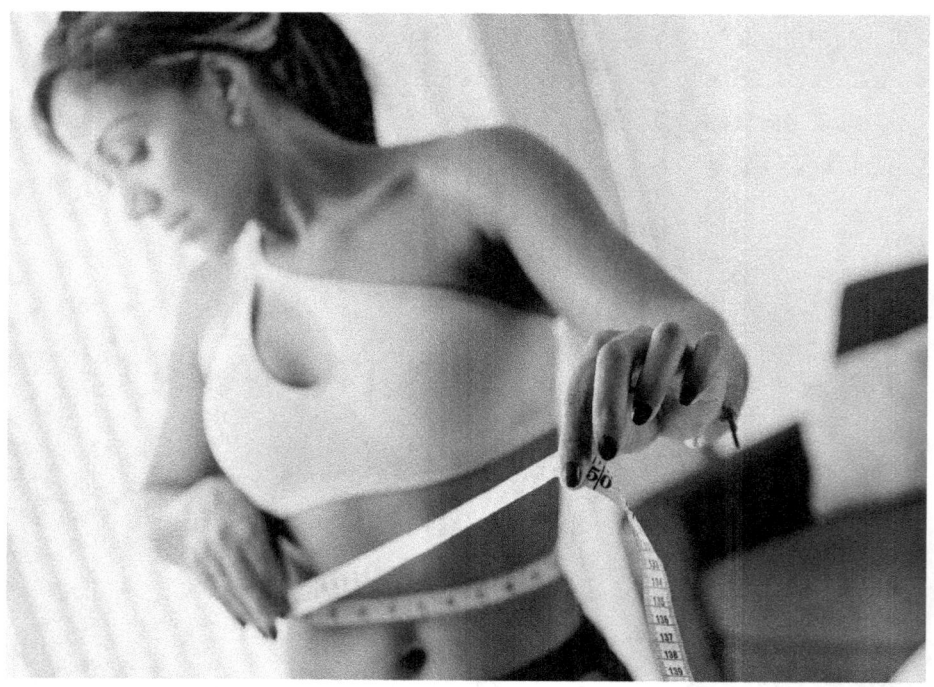

WEIGHT LOSS JOURNAL

WHAT IS MY
IDEAL WEIGHT?

WHAT ACTIVITIES &
EXERCISES WILL I
DO TO GET MYSELF
INTO SHAPE?

WHAT HEALTHY
FOODS DO I NEED TO
INCORPORATE INTO
MY DIET?

WHAT JUNK FOODS
DO I NEED TO
ELIMINATE FROM MY
DIET?

WHO WILL I CALL
TO SUPPORT ME
AND KEEP ME
ACCOUNTABLE?

WEIGHT LOSS ANNUAL

YEAR : _____

	Start	End	Gain	Loss	NOTES
JANUARY					
WK 1	_____	_____	○	○	
WK 2	_____	_____	○	○	
WK 3	_____	_____	○	○	
WK 4	_____	_____	○	○	

	Start	End	Gain	Loss	NOTES
FEBRUARY					
WK 1	_____	_____	○	○	
WK 2	_____	_____	○	○	
WK 3	_____	_____	○	○	
WK 4	_____	_____	○	○	

	Start	End	Gain	Loss	NOTES
MARCH					
WK 1	_____	_____	○	○	
WK 2	_____	_____	○	○	
WK 3	_____	_____	○	○	
WK 4	_____	_____	○	○	

	Start	End	Gain	Loss	NOTES
APRIL					
WK 1	_____	_____	○	○	
WK 2	_____	_____	○	○	
WK 3	_____	_____	○	○	
WK 4	_____	_____	○	○	

WEIGHT LOSS ANNUAL

YEAR : _____

MAY

	Start	End	Gain	Loss
WK 1	_____	_____	○	○
WK 2	_____	_____	○	○
WK 3	_____	_____	○	○
WK 4	_____	_____	○	○

NOTES

JUNE

	Start	End	Gain	Loss
WK 1	_____	_____	○	○
WK 2	_____	_____	○	○
WK 3	_____	_____	○	○
WK 4	_____	_____	○	○

NOTES

JULY

	Start	End	Gain	Loss
WK 1	_____	_____	○	○
WK 2	_____	_____	○	○
WK 3	_____	_____	○	○
WK 4	_____	_____	○	○

NOTES

AUGUST

	Start	End	Gain	Loss
WK 1	_____	_____	○	○
WK 2	_____	_____	○	○
WK 3	_____	_____	○	○
WK 4	_____	_____	○	○

NOTES

WEIGHT LOSS ANNUAL

YEAR : _____

SEPTEMBER

	Start	End	Gain	Loss
WK 1	_____	_____	○	○
WK 2	_____	_____	○	○
WK 3	_____	_____	○	○
WK 4	_____	_____	○	○

NOTES

OCTOBER

	Start	End	Gain	Loss
WK 1	_____	_____	○	○
WK 2	_____	_____	○	○
WK 3	_____	_____	○	○
WK 4	_____	_____	○	○

NOTES

NOVEMBER

	Start	End	Gain	Loss
WK 1	_____	_____	○	○
WK 2	_____	_____	○	○
WK 3	_____	_____	○	○
WK 4	_____	_____	○	○

NOTES

DECEMBER

	Start	End	Gain	Loss
WK 1	_____	_____	○	○
WK 2	_____	_____	○	○
WK 3	_____	_____	○	○
WK 4	_____	_____	○	○

NOTES

DIET LOG

DATE:

CALORIES	CARBS (g)	SUGAR (g)	PROTEIN (g)	FAT (g)

Time	Food	Calories	Carbs	Sugar	Protein	Fat
Total						

DIET LOG

DATE: _____

CALORIES	CARBS (g)	SUGAR (g)	PROTEIN (g)	FAT (g)

Time	Food	Calories	Carbs	Sugar	Protein	Fat
Total						

DIET LOG

DATE:

CALORIES	CARBS (g)	SUGAR (g)	PROTEIN (g)	FAT (g)

Time	Food	Calories	Carbs	Sugar	Protein	Fat
Total						

DIET LOG

DATE: _____

CALORIES	CARBS (g)	SUGAR (g)	PROTEIN (g)	FAT (g)

Time	Food	Calories	Carbs	Sugar	Protein	Fat
Total						

DIET LOG

DATE: _____

CALORIES	CARBS (g)	SUGAR (g)	PROTEIN (g)	FAT (g)

Time	Food	Calories	Carbs	Sugar	Protein	Fat
Total						

DIET LOG

DATE: _____

CALORIES	CARBS (g)	SUGAR (g)	PROTEIN (g)	FAT (g)

Time	Food	Calories	Carbs	Sugar	Protein	Fat
Total						

DIET LOG

DATE:

CALORIES	CARBS (g)	SUGAR (g)	PROTEIN (g)	FAT (g)

Time	Food	Calories	Carbs	Sugar	Protein	Fat
Total						

INTERMITTENT FASTING

MONTH:

	MONDAY

GOAL	12	1	2	3	4	5	6	7	8	9	10	11	12	1	2	3	4	5	6	7	8	9	10	11
ACTUAL	12	1	2	3	4	5	6	7	8	9	10	11	12	1	2	3	4	5	6	7	8	9	10	11

	TUESDAY

GOAL	12	1	2	3	4	5	6	7	8	9	10	11	12	1	2	3	4	5	6	7	8	9	10	11
ACTUAL	12	1	2	3	4	5	6	7	8	9	10	11	12	1	2	3	4	5	6	7	8	9	10	11

	WEDNESDAY

GOAL	12	1	2	3	4	5	6	7	8	9	10	11	12	1	2	3	4	5	6	7	8	9	10	11
ACTUAL	12	1	2	3	4	5	6	7	8	9	10	11	12	1	2	3	4	5	6	7	8	9	10	11

	THURSDAY

GOAL	12	1	2	3	4	5	6	7	8	9	10	11	12	1	2	3	4	5	6	7	8	9	10	11
ACTUAL	12	1	2	3	4	5	6	7	8	9	10	11	12	1	2	3	4	5	6	7	8	9	10	11

	FRIDAY

GOAL	12	1	2	3	4	5	6	7	8	9	10	11	12	1	2	3	4	5	6	7	8	9	10	11
ACTUAL	12	1	2	3	4	5	6	7	8	9	10	11	12	1	2	3	4	5	6	7	8	9	10	11

	SATURDAY

GOAL	12	1	2	3	4	5	6	7	8	9	10	11	12	1	2	3	4	5	6	7	8	9	10	11
ACTUAL	12	1	2	3	4	5	6	7	8	9	10	11	12	1	2	3	4	5	6	7	8	9	10	11

	SUNDAY

GOAL	12	1	2	3	4	5	6	7	8	9	10	11	12	1	2	3	4	5	6	7	8	9	10	11
ACTUAL	12	1	2	3	4	5	6	7	8	9	10	11	12	1	2	3	4	5	6	7	8	9	10	11

INTERMITTENT FASTING

MONTH:

_____

MONDAY

	12	1	2	3	4	5	6	7	8	9	10	11	12	1	2	3	4	5	6	7	8	9	10	11
GOAL	12	1	2	3	4	5	6	7	8	9	10	11	12	1	2	3	4	5	6	7	8	9	10	11
ACTUAL	12	1	2	3	4	5	6	7	8	9	10	11	12	1	2	3	4	5	6	7	8	9	10	11

TUESDAY

	12	1	2	3	4	5	6	7	8	9	10	11	12	1	2	3	4	5	6	7	8	9	10	11
GOAL	12	1	2	3	4	5	6	7	8	9	10	11	12	1	2	3	4	5	6	7	8	9	10	11
ACTUAL	12	1	2	3	4	5	6	7	8	9	10	11	12	1	2	3	4	5	6	7	8	9	10	11

WEDNESDAY

	12	1	2	3	4	5	6	7	8	9	10	11	12	1	2	3	4	5	6	7	8	9	10	11
GOAL	12	1	2	3	4	5	6	7	8	9	10	11	12	1	2	3	4	5	6	7	8	9	10	11
ACTUAL	12	1	2	3	4	5	6	7	8	9	10	11	12	1	2	3	4	5	6	7	8	9	10	11

THURSDAY

	12	1	2	3	4	5	6	7	8	9	10	11	12	1	2	3	4	5	6	7	8	9	10	11
GOAL	12	1	2	3	4	5	6	7	8	9	10	11	12	1	2	3	4	5	6	7	8	9	10	11
ACTUAL	12	1	2	3	4	5	6	7	8	9	10	11	12	1	2	3	4	5	6	7	8	9	10	11

FRIDAY

	12	1	2	3	4	5	6	7	8	9	10	11	12	1	2	3	4	5	6	7	8	9	10	11
GOAL	12	1	2	3	4	5	6	7	8	9	10	11	12	1	2	3	4	5	6	7	8	9	10	11
ACTUAL	12	1	2	3	4	5	6	7	8	9	10	11	12	1	2	3	4	5	6	7	8	9	10	11

SATURDAY

	12	1	2	3	4	5	6	7	8	9	10	11	12	1	2	3	4	5	6	7	8	9	10	11
GOAL	12	1	2	3	4	5	6	7	8	9	10	11	12	1	2	3	4	5	6	7	8	9	10	11
ACTUAL	12	1	2	3	4	5	6	7	8	9	10	11	12	1	2	3	4	5	6	7	8	9	10	11

SUNDAY

	12	1	2	3	4	5	6	7	8	9	10	11	12	1	2	3	4	5	6	7	8	9	10	11
GOAL	12	1	2	3	4	5	6	7	8	9	10	11	12	1	2	3	4	5	6	7	8	9	10	11
ACTUAL	12	1	2	3	4	5	6	7	8	9	10	11	12	1	2	3	4	5	6	7	8	9	10	11

INTERMITTENT FASTING

MONTH:

MONDAY

GOAL	12	1	2	3	4	5	6	7	8	9	10	11	12	1	2	3	4	5	6	7	8	9	10	11
ACTUAL	12	1	2	3	4	5	6	7	8	9	10	11	12	1	2	3	4	5	6	7	8	9	10	11

TUESDAY

GOAL	12	1	2	3	4	5	6	7	8	9	10	11	12	1	2	3	4	5	6	7	8	9	10	11
ACTUAL	12	1	2	3	4	5	6	7	8	9	10	11	12	1	2	3	4	5	6	7	8	9	10	11

WEDNESDAY

GOAL	12	1	2	3	4	5	6	7	8	9	10	11	12	1	2	3	4	5	6	7	8	9	10	11
ACTUAL	12	1	2	3	4	5	6	7	8	9	10	11	12	1	2	3	4	5	6	7	8	9	10	11

THURSDAY

GOAL	12	1	2	3	4	5	6	7	8	9	10	11	12	1	2	3	4	5	6	7	8	9	10	11
ACTUAL	12	1	2	3	4	5	6	7	8	9	10	11	12	1	2	3	4	5	6	7	8	9	10	11

FRIDAY

GOAL	12	1	2	3	4	5	6	7	8	9	10	11	12	1	2	3	4	5	6	7	8	9	10	11
ACTUAL	12	1	2	3	4	5	6	7	8	9	10	11	12	1	2	3	4	5	6	7	8	9	10	11

SATURDAY

GOAL	12	1	2	3	4	5	6	7	8	9	10	11	12	1	2	3	4	5	6	7	8	9	10	11
ACTUAL	12	1	2	3	4	5	6	7	8	9	10	11	12	1	2	3	4	5	6	7	8	9	10	11

SUNDAY

GOAL	12	1	2	3	4	5	6	7	8	9	10	11	12	1	2	3	4	5	6	7	8	9	10	11
ACTUAL	12	1	2	3	4	5	6	7	8	9	10	11	12	1	2	3	4	5	6	7	8	9	10	11

WEIGHT LOSS GOAL

Notes:

LBS

100%

LBS

90%

LBS

80%

LBS

70%

LBS

60%

LBS

50%

LBS

40%

LBS

30%

LBS

20%

LBS

10%

LBS

START

WEIGHT LOSS GOALS

Start Date:	Target Date:

Goal: _____

_____

_____

_____

Why: _____

_____

_____

Measurements:

	Weight	Neck	Chest	Waist	Hips	Thighs	Bust	Biceps
Start								
After								

Actions to Achieve Goal:

_____

_____

_____

_____

_____

_____

_____

_____

_____

_____

_____

_____

_____

_____

_____

_____

_____

Rewards:

_____

_____

_____

_____

_____

_____

_____

_____

_____

_____

_____

_____

_____

WEIGHT LOSS GOALS

Start Date:	Target Date:

Goal: _____

_____

_____

_____

Why: _____

_____

_____

_____

Measurements:

	Weight	Neck	Chest	Waist	Hips	Thighs	Bust	Biceps
Start								
After								

Actions to Achieve Goal:

_____

_____

_____

_____

_____

_____

_____

_____

_____

_____

_____

_____

_____

_____

_____

_____

Rewards:

_____

_____

_____

_____

_____

_____

_____

_____

_____

_____

_____

WEIGHT LOSS GOALS

Start Date:	Target Date:

Goal: _____   Why: _____
_____   _____
_____   _____
_____

Measurements:

	Weight	Neck	Chest	Waist	Hips	Thighs	Bust	Biceps
Start								
After								

Actions to Achieve Goal: Rewards:

WEIGHT LOSS GOALS

Start Date:	Target Date:

Goal: _____
_____
_____

Why: _____
_____
_____

Measurements:

	Weight	Neck	Chest	Waist	Hips	Thighs	Bust	Biceps
Start								
After								

Actions to Achieve Goal:

_____
_____
_____
_____
_____
_____
_____
_____
_____
_____
_____
_____
_____
_____

Rewards:

_____
_____
_____
_____
_____
_____
_____
_____
_____
_____

WEIGHT LOSS GOALS

Start Date:	Target Date:

Goal: _____
_____
_____
_____

Why: _____
_____
_____

Measurements:

	Weight	Neck	Chest	Waist	Hips	Thighs	Bust	Biceps
Start								
After								

Actions to Achieve Goal:

_____
_____
_____
_____
_____
_____
_____
_____
_____
_____
_____
_____
_____
_____

Rewards:

_____
_____
_____
_____
_____
_____
_____
_____
_____
_____
_____

WEIGHT LOSS GOALS

Start Date:	Target Date:

Goal: _____
_____
_____
_____

Why: _____
_____
_____
_____

Measurements:

	Weight	Neck	Chest	Waist	Hips	Thighs	Bust	Biceps
Start								
After								

Actions to Achieve Goal:

_____
_____
_____
_____
_____
_____
_____
_____
_____
_____
_____
_____
_____
_____

Rewards:

_____
_____
_____
_____
_____
_____
_____
_____
_____
_____
_____
_____

WEIGHT LOSS GOALS

Start Date:	Target Date:

Goal: _____

_____

_____

_____

Why: _____

_____

_____

Measurements:

	Weight	Neck	Chest	Waist	Hips	Thighs	Bust	Biceps
Start								
After								

Actions to Achieve Goal:

_____

_____

_____

_____

_____

_____

_____

_____

_____

_____

_____

_____

_____

_____

_____

_____

Rewards:

_____

_____

_____

_____

_____

_____

_____

_____

_____

_____

_____

_____

BEFORE & AFTER

TOP
GOAL —————————————————————

BEFORE
DATE ————————————

AFTER
DATE ————————————

MEASUREMENTS

CHEST		CHEST	
WAIST		WAIST	
HIP		HIP	
ARMS		ARMS	
THIGHS		THIGHS	

NUMBERS

WEIGHT		WEIGHT	
BMI		BMI	
BODY FAT		BODY FAT	
MUSCLE		MUSCLE	

MOTIVATION

NEXT STEPS

BEFORE & AFTER

TOP
GOAL ————————————————————

BEFORE   AFTER
DATE ————————————   DATE ————————————

MEASUREMENTS

CHEST		CHEST	
WAIST		WAIST	
HIP		HIP	
ARMS		ARMS	
THIGHS		THIGHS	

NUMBERS

WEIGHT   WEIGHT

BMI   BMI

BODY FAT   BODY FAT

MUSCLE   MUSCLE

MOTIVATION   NEXT STEPS

BEFORE & AFTER

TOP
GOAL _____

BEFORE
DATE _____

AFTER
DATE _____

MEASUREMENTS

CHEST		CHEST	
WAIST		WAIST	
HIP		HIP	
ARMS		ARMS	
THIGHS		THIGHS	

NUMBERS

WEIGHT		WEIGHT	
BMI		BMI	
BODY FAT		BODY FAT	
MUSCLE		MUSCLE	

MOTIVATION

NEXT STEPS

BEFORE & AFTER

TOP
GOAL ————————————————————————

BEFORE
DATE ————————————————

AFTER
DATE ————————————————

MEASUREMENTS

CHEST		CHEST	
WAIST		WAIST	
HIP		HIP	
ARMS		ARMS	
THIGHS		THIGHS	

NUMBERS

WEIGHT

BMI

BODY FAT

MUSCLE

WEIGHT

BMI

BODY FAT

MUSCLE

MOTIVATION

NEXT STEPS

BEFORE & AFTER

START DATE:	FINISH DATE:
BEFORE:	AFTER:

BEFORE		AFTER	
NECK		NECK	
BICEP L		BICEP L	
BICEP R		BICEP R	
CHEST		CHEST	
WAIST		WAIST	
HIPS		HIPS	
TIGHT L		TIGHT L	
TIGHT R		TIGHT R	
WEIGHT		WEIGHT	

BEFORE & AFTER

START DATE:	FINISH DATE:
BEFORE:	AFTER:

BEFORE		AFTER	
NECK		NECK	
BICEP L		BICEP L	
BICEP R		BICEP R	
CHEST		CHEST	
WAIST		WAIST	
HIPS		HIPS	
TIGHT L		TIGHT L	
TIGHT R		TIGHT R	
WEIGHT		WEIGHT	

BEFORE & AFTER

START DATE:	FINISH DATE:
BEFORE:	AFTER:

BEFORE		AFTER	
NECK		NECK	
BICEP L		BICEP L	
BICEP R		BICEP R	
CHEST		CHEST	
WAIST		WAIST	
HIPS		HIPS	
TIGHT L		TIGHT L	
TIGHT R		TIGHT R	
WEIGHT		WEIGHT	

BEFORE & AFTER

START DATE:	FINISH DATE:
BEFORE:	AFTER:

BEFORE		AFTER	
NECK		NECK	
BICEP L		BICEP L	
BICEP R		BICEP R	
CHEST		CHEST	
WAIST		WAIST	
HIPS		HIPS	
TIGHT L		TIGHT L	
TIGHT R		TIGHT R	
WEIGHT		WEIGHT	

WEIGHT LOSS TRACKER

MONTH _____

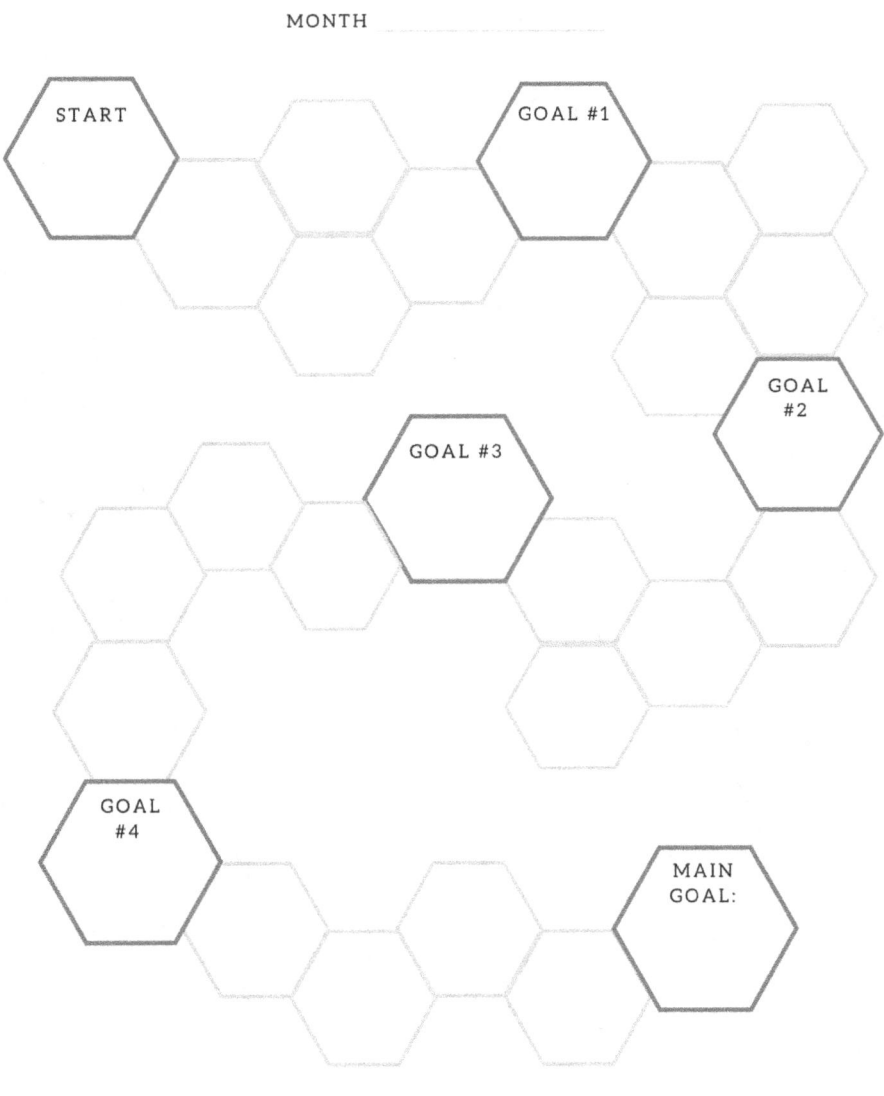

START

GOAL #1

GOAL #2

GOAL #3

GOAL #4

MAIN GOAL:

GOALS		REWARDS	
#1			
#2			
#3			
#4			
MAIN:			

WEIGHT LOSS TRACKER

MONTH

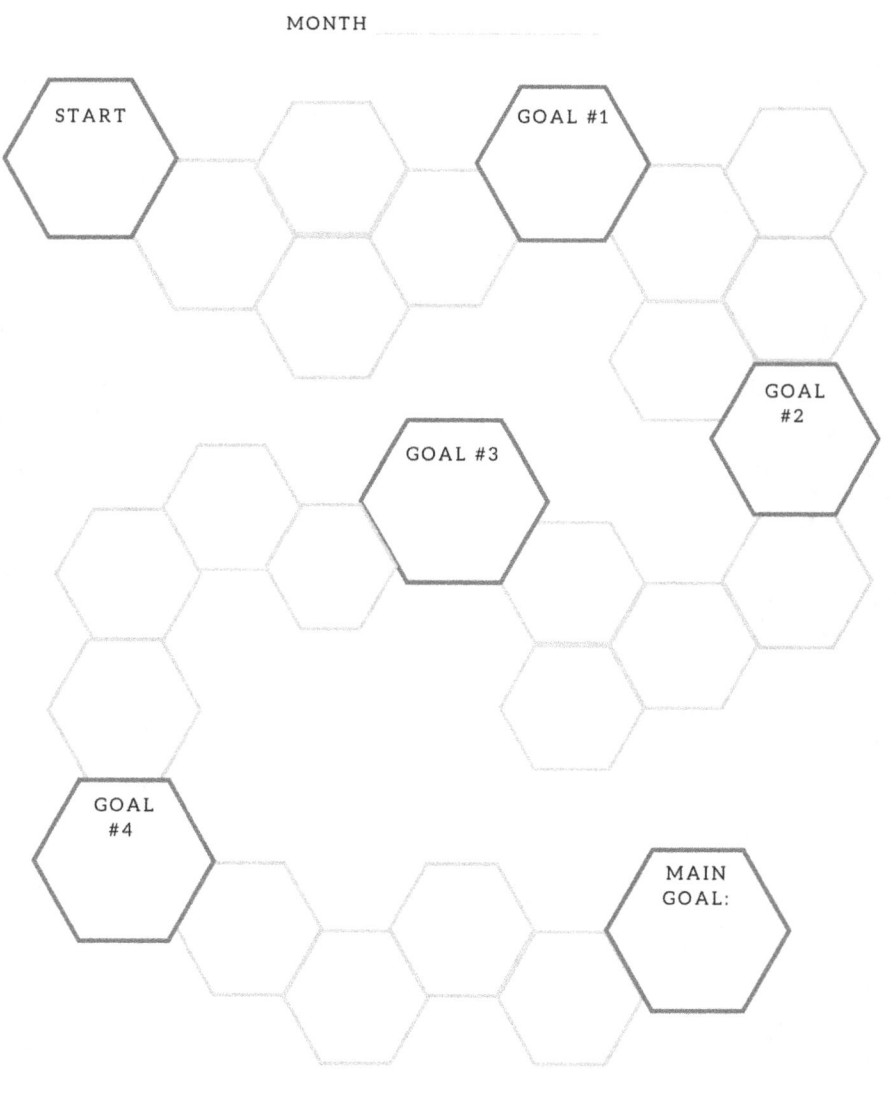

START

GOAL #1

GOAL #2

GOAL #3

GOAL #4

MAIN GOAL:

GOALS
#1
#2
#3
#4
MAIN:

REWARDS

WEIGHT LOSS TRACKER

MONTH _____

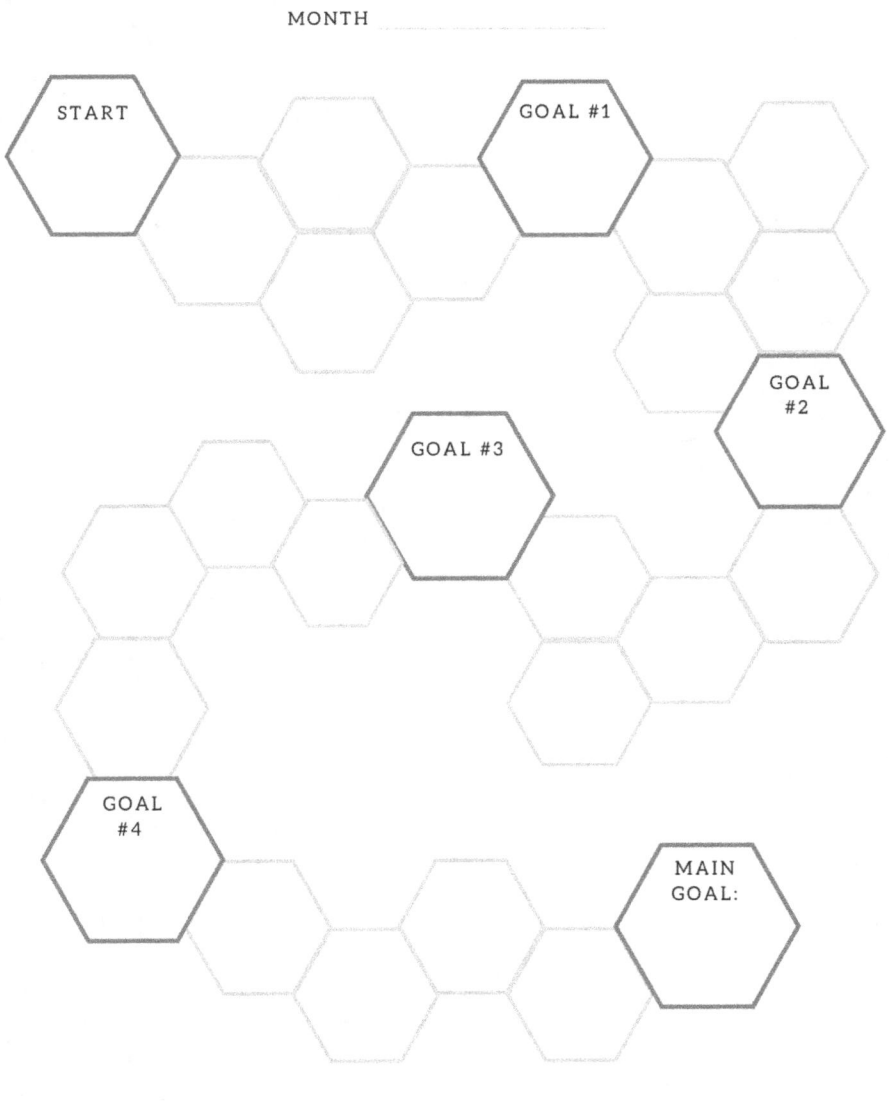

START

GOAL #1

GOAL #2

GOAL #3

GOAL #4

MAIN GOAL:

GOALS		REWARDS	
#1			
#2			
#3			
#4			
MAIN:			

WEIGHT LOSS TRACKER

MONTH _____

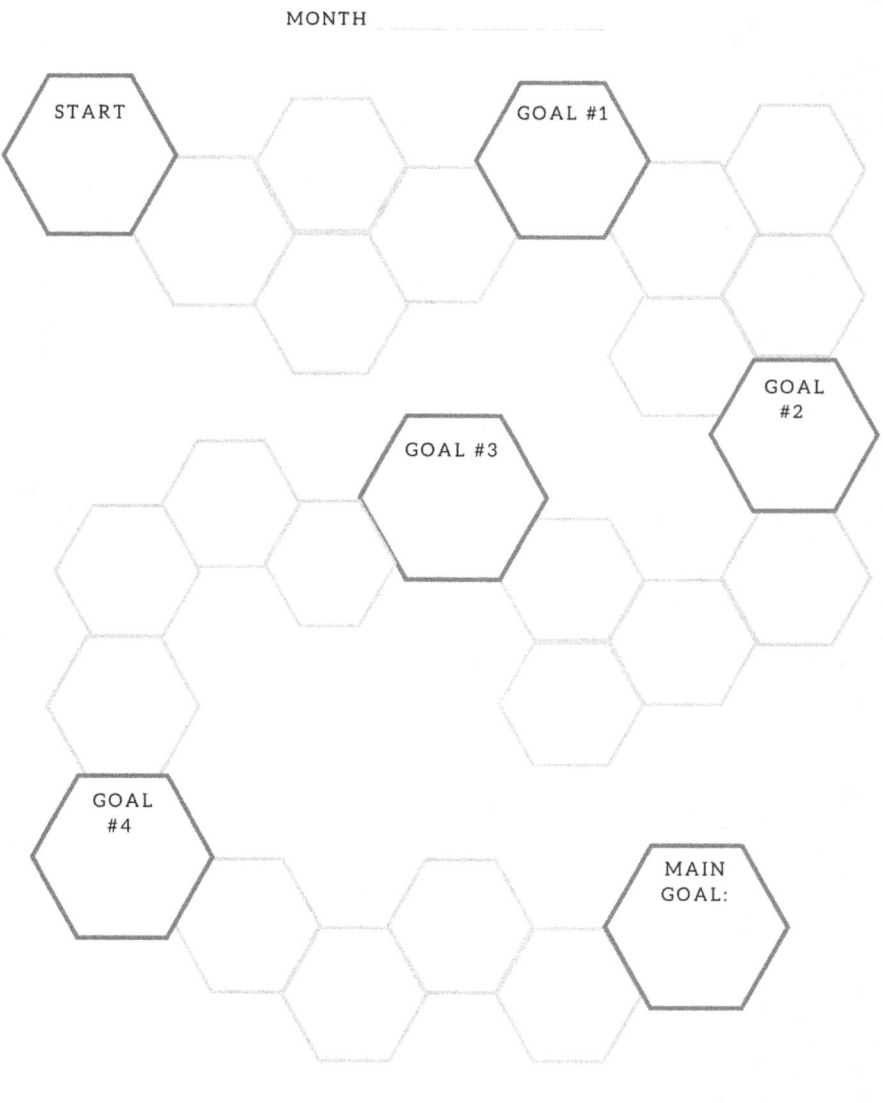

START

GOAL #1

GOAL #2

GOAL #3

GOAL #4

MAIN GOAL:

GOALS		REWARDS	
#1			
#2			
#3			
#4			
MAIN:			

WEIGHT LOSS TRACKER

MONTH

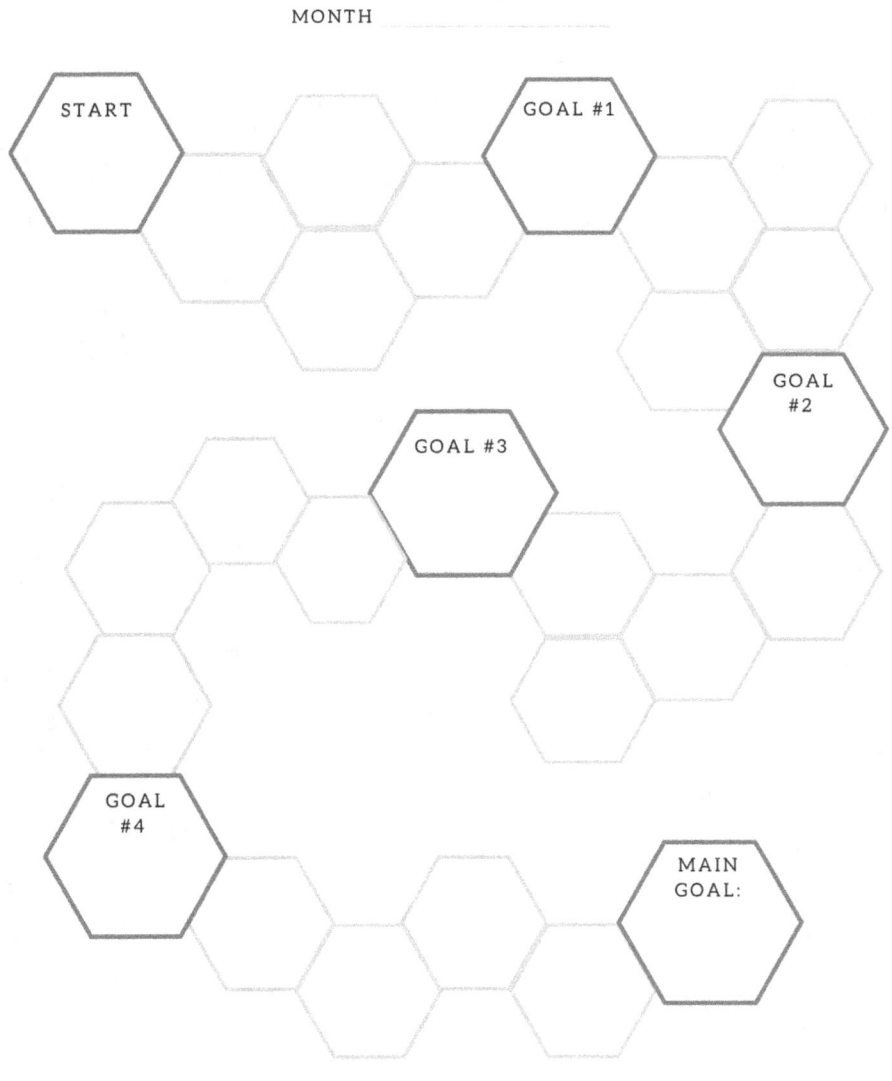

START

GOAL #1

GOAL #2

GOAL #3

GOAL #4

MAIN GOAL:

GOALS
#1
#2
#3
#4
MAIN:

REWARDS

WEIGHT LOSS TRACKER

MONTH

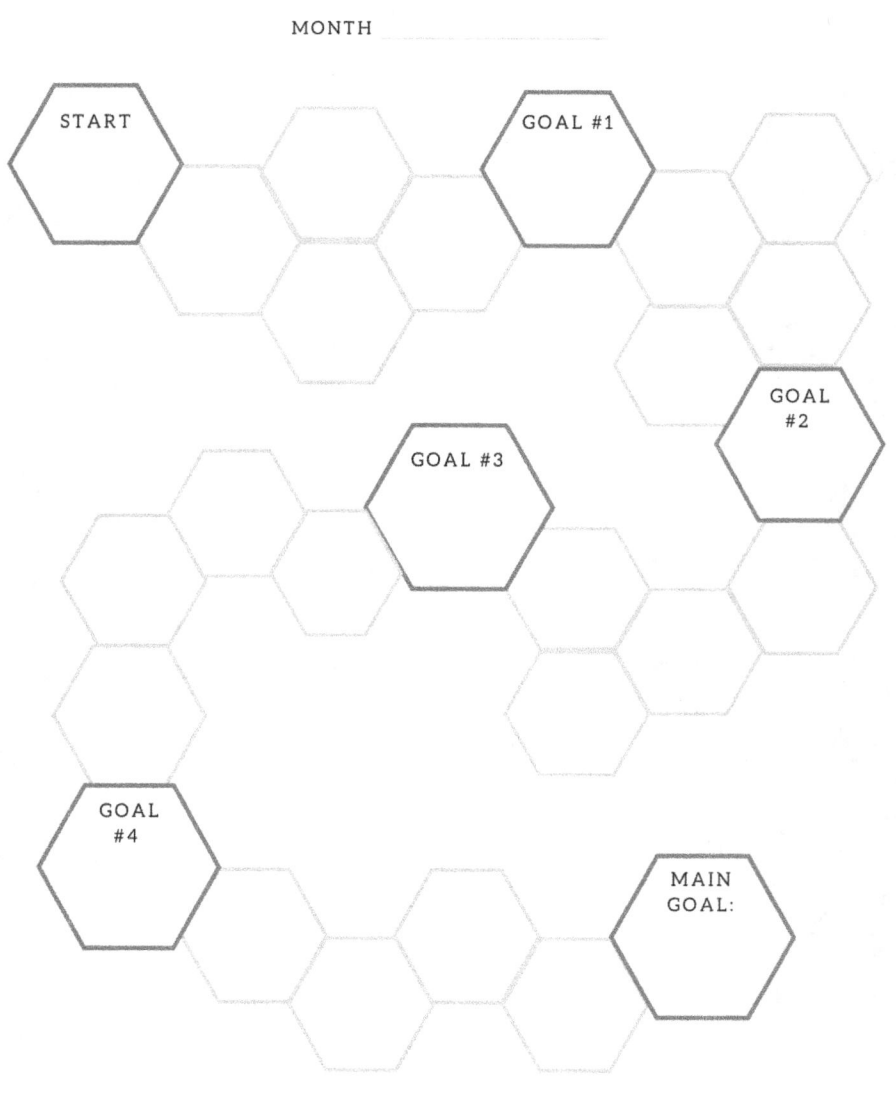

START

GOAL #1

GOAL #2

GOAL #3

GOAL #4

MAIN GOAL:

GOALS		REWARDS	
	#1		
	#2		
	#3		
	#4		
	MAIN:		

MEASUREMENT TRACKER

	Weight	Neck	Chest	Waist	Hips	Thighs	Bust	Biceps
January								
February								
March								
April								
May								
June								
July								
August								
September								
October								
November								
December								

Notes

MEASUREMENT TRACKER

DATE:

GOAL

PROGRESS

	Week 01	Week 02	Week 03	Week 04	Week 05	Week 06	Week 07	Week 08
WEIGHT								
NECK								
CHEST								
ARMS								
WAIST								
HIPS								
THIGHS								
CALF								

NOTES

MEASUREMENT TRACKER

DATE:

GOAL

PROGRESS							
Week 01	Week 02	Week 03	Week 04	Week 05	Week 06	Week 07	Week 08

WEIGHT

NECK

CHEST

ARMS

WAIST

HIPS

THIGHS

CALF

NOTES

MEASUREMENT TRACKER

DATE:

GOAL

PROGRESS

	Week 01	Week 02	Week 03	Week 04	Week 05	Week 06	Week 07	Week 08
WEIGHT								
NECK								
CHEST								
ARMS								
WAIST								
HIPS								
THIGHS								
CALF								

NOTES

MEASUREMENT TRACKER

DATE:

GOAL

	PROGRESS							
	Week 01	Week 02	Week 03	Week 04	Week 05	Week 06	Week 07	Week 08
WEIGHT								
NECK								
CHEST								
ARMS								
WAIST								
HIPS								
THIGHS								
CALF								

NOTES

HEALTHY RECIPE

Name:

Prep Time: Cooking Time: Servings:

Ingredients

Rating: ☆☆☆☆☆

- ○
- ○
- ○
- ○
- ○
- ○
- ○
- ○
- ○
- ○
- ○

- ○
- ○
- ○
- ○
- ○
- ○
- ○
- ○
- ○

Instructions

HEALTHY RECIPE

Name:

Prep Time: Cooking Time: Servings:

Ingredients

Rating: ☆☆☆☆☆

- ○
- ○
- ○
- ○
- ○
- ○
- ○
- ○
- ○
- ○
- ○

- ○
- ○
- ○
- ○
- ○
- ○
- ○
- ○
- ○
- ○

Instructions

HEALTHY RECIPE

Name:

Prep Time:

Cooking Time:

Servings:

Ingredients

Rating: ☆☆☆☆☆

- ○
- ○
- ○
- ○
- ○
- ○
- ○
- ○
- ○
- ○
- ○

- ○
- ○
- ○
- ○
- ○
- ○
- ○
- ○
- ○
- ○
- ○

Instructions

HEALTHY RECIPE

Name:

Prep Time: Cooking Time: Servings:

Ingredients

Rating: ☆☆☆☆☆

- ○
- ○
- ○
- ○
- ○
- ○
- ○
- ○
- ○
- ○

- ○
- ○
- ○
- ○
- ○
- ○
- ○
- ○
- ○
- ○

Instructions

HEALTHY RECIPE

Name:

Prep Time: .... Cooking Time: .... Servings: ....

Ingredients

Rating: ☆☆☆☆☆

- ○ ....
- ○ ....
- ○ ....
- ○ ....
- ○ ....
- ○ ....
- ○ ....
- ○ ....
- ○ ....
- ○ ....
- ○ ....

- ○ ....
- ○ ....
- ○ ....
- ○ ....
- ○ ....
- ○ ....
- ○ ....
- ○ ....
- ○ ....
- ○ ....

Instructions

....
....
....
....
....
....
....
....
....

HEALTHY RECIPE

Name:

Prep Time: Cooking Time: Servings:

Ingredients   Rating: ☆☆☆☆☆

- ○
- ○
- ○
- ○
- ○
- ○
- ○
- ○
- ○
- ○

- ○
- ○
- ○
- ○
- ○
- ○
- ○
- ○
- ○
- ○

Instructions

HEALTHY RECIPE

Name:

Prep Time: Cooking Time: Servings:

Ingredients   Rating: ☆☆☆☆☆

- ○
- ○
- ○
- ○
- ○
- ○
- ○
- ○
- ○
- ○
- ○

- ○
- ○
- ○
- ○
- ○
- ○
- ○
- ○
- ○
- ○

Instructions

HEALTHY RECIPE

Name:

Prep Time:

Cooking Time:

Servings:

Ingredients

Rating: ☆☆☆☆☆

- ○
- ○
- ○
- ○
- ○
- ○
- ○
- ○
- ○
- ○
- ○

- ○
- ○
- ○
- ○
- ○
- ○
- ○
- ○
- ○
- ○

Instructions

HEALTHY RECIPE

Name:

Prep Time: Cooking Time: Servings:

Ingredients   Rating: ☆☆☆☆☆

- ○
- ○
- ○
- ○
- ○
- ○
- ○
- ○
- ○
- ○

- ○
- ○
- ○
- ○
- ○
- ○
- ○
- ○
- ○
- ○

Instructions

HEALTHY RECIPE

Name:

Prep Time:

Cooking Time:

Servings:

Ingredients

Rating: ☆☆☆☆☆

- ○
- ○
- ○
- ○
- ○
- ○
- ○
- ○
- ○
- ○

- ○
- ○
- ○
- ○
- ○
- ○
- ○
- ○
- ○
- ○

Instructions

HEALTHY RECIPE

Name:

Prep Time: Cooking Time: Servings:

Ingredients

Rating: ☆☆☆☆☆

- ○
- ○
- ○
- ○
- ○
- ○
- ○
- ○
- ○
- ○
- ○

- ○
- ○
- ○
- ○
- ○
- ○
- ○
- ○
- ○
- ○
- ○

Instructions

RECIPE PLANNER

Category:

Prep Time:

Cook Time:

Total Time:

Servings:

Difficulty: ☐ ☐ ☐ ☐ ☐

Source:

Total Needed:

Prep Ahead:

Notes:

Name:

Ingredients:

Directions:

RECIPE PLANNER

Category:

Prep Time:

Cook Time:

Total Time:

Servings:

Difficulty: ☐ ☐ ☐ ☐

Source:

Total Needed:

Prep Ahead:

Notes:

Name:

Ingredients:

Directions:

RECIPE PLANNER

Category:

Prep Time:

Cook Time:

Total Time:

Servings:

Difficulty: ☐ ☐ ☐ ☐ ☐

Source:

Total Needed:

Prep Ahead:

Notes:

Name:

Ingredients:

Directions:

RECIPE PLANNER

Category:

Prep Time:

Cook Time:

Total Time:

Servings:

Difficulty: ☐ ☐ ☐ ☐ ☐

Source:

Total Needed:

Prep Ahead:

Notes:

Name:

Ingredients:

Directions:

RECIPE PLANNER

Category:

Prep Time:

Cook Time:

Total Time:

Servings:

Difficulty: ☐ ☐ ☐ ☐ ☐

Source:

Total Needed:

Prep Ahead:

Notes:

Name:

Ingredients:

Directions:

RECIPE PLANNER

Category:

Prep Time:

Cook Time:

Total Time:

Servings:

Difficulty: ☐ ☐ ☐ ☐ ☐

Source:

Total Needed:

Prep Ahead:

Notes:

Name:

Ingredients:

Directions:

RECIPE PLANNER

Category:

Prep Time:

Cook Time:

Total Time:

Servings:

Difficulty: ☐ ☐ ☐ ☐ ☐

Source:

Total Needed:

Prep Ahead:

Notes:

Name:

Ingredients:

Directions:

RECIPE PLANNER

Category:

Prep Time:

Cook Time:

Total Time:

Servings:

Difficulty: ☐ ☐ ☐ ☐ ☐

Source:

Total Needed:

Prep Ahead:

Notes:

Name:

Ingredients:

Directions:

RECIPE PLANNER

Category:

Name:

Prep Time:

Ingredients:

Cook Time:

Total Time:

Servings:

Difficulty: ☐ ☐ ☐ ☐ ☐

Source:

Directions:

Total Needed:

Prep Ahead:

Notes:

FAVOURITE RECIPES

Date:

Recipe Name	Difficulty	Raiting
	1 2 3 4 5	☆☆☆☆☆
	1 2 3 4 5	☆☆☆☆☆
	1 2 3 4 5	☆☆☆☆☆
	1 2 3 4 5	☆☆☆☆☆
	1 2 3 4 5	☆☆☆☆☆
	1 2 3 4 5	☆☆☆☆☆
	1 2 3 4 5	☆☆☆☆☆
	1 2 3 4 5	☆☆☆☆☆
	1 2 3 4 5	☆☆☆☆☆
	1 2 3 4 5	☆☆☆☆☆
	1 2 3 4 5	☆☆☆☆☆
	1 2 3 4 5	☆☆☆☆☆
	1 2 3 4 5	☆☆☆☆☆

FAVOURITE RECIPES

Date:

Recipe Name	Difficulty	Raiting
	1 2 3 4 5	☆☆☆☆☆
	1 2 3 4 5	☆☆☆☆☆
	1 2 3 4 5	☆☆☆☆☆
	1 2 3 4 5	☆☆☆☆☆
	1 2 3 4 5	☆☆☆☆☆
	1 2 3 4 5	☆☆☆☆☆
	1 2 3 4 5	☆☆☆☆☆
	1 2 3 4 5	☆☆☆☆☆
	1 2 3 4 5	☆☆☆☆☆
	1 2 3 4 5	☆☆☆☆☆
	1 2 3 4 5	☆☆☆☆☆
	1 2 3 4 5	☆☆☆☆☆
	1 2 3 4 5	☆☆☆☆☆

FAVOURITE RECIPES

Date:

Recipe Name	Difficulty	Raiting
	1 2 3 4 5	☆☆☆☆☆
	1 2 3 4 5	☆☆☆☆☆
	1 2 3 4 5	☆☆☆☆☆
	1 2 3 4 5	☆☆☆☆☆
	1 2 3 4 5	☆☆☆☆☆
	1 2 3 4 5	☆☆☆☆☆
	1 2 3 4 5	☆☆☆☆☆
	1 2 3 4 5	☆☆☆☆☆
	1 2 3 4 5	☆☆☆☆☆
	1 2 3 4 5	☆☆☆☆☆
	1 2 3 4 5	☆☆☆☆☆
	1 2 3 4 5	☆☆☆☆☆
	1 2 3 4 5	☆☆☆☆☆

FAVOURITE RECIPES

Date:

Recipe Name	Difficulty	Raiting
	1 2 3 4 5	☆☆☆☆☆
	1 2 3 4 5	☆☆☆☆☆
	1 2 3 4 5	☆☆☆☆☆
	1 2 3 4 5	☆☆☆☆☆
	1 2 3 4 5	☆☆☆☆☆
	1 2 3 4 5	☆☆☆☆☆
	1 2 3 4 5	☆☆☆☆☆
	1 2 3 4 5	☆☆☆☆☆
	1 2 3 4 5	☆☆☆☆☆
	1 2 3 4 5	☆☆☆☆☆
	1 2 3 4 5	☆☆☆☆☆
	1 2 3 4 5	☆☆☆☆☆
	1 2 3 4 5	☆☆☆☆☆

FAVOURITE RECIPES

Date:

Recipe Name	Difficulty	Raiting
	1 2 3 4 5	☆☆☆☆☆
	1 2 3 4 5	☆☆☆☆☆
	1 2 3 4 5	☆☆☆☆☆
	1 2 3 4 5	☆☆☆☆☆
	1 2 3 4 5	☆☆☆☆☆
	1 2 3 4 5	☆☆☆☆☆
	1 2 3 4 5	☆☆☆☆☆
	1 2 3 4 5	☆☆☆☆☆
	1 2 3 4 5	☆☆☆☆☆
	1 2 3 4 5	☆☆☆☆☆
	1 2 3 4 5	☆☆☆☆☆
	1 2 3 4 5	☆☆☆☆☆
	1 2 3 4 5	☆☆☆☆☆

MEAL PLANNER

WEEK _____

Day	Breakfast	Lunch	Dinner	Dessert
M				
T				
W				
T				
F				
S				
S				

Cheeky Treats & Snacks:

MEAL PLANNER

WEEK _____

Day	Breakfast	Lunch	Dinner	Dessert
M				
T				
W				
T				
F				
S				
S				

Cheeky Treats & Snacks:

MEAL PLANNER

WEEK _____

Day	Breakfast	Lunch	Dinner	Dessert
M				
T				
W				
T				
F				
S				
S				

Cheeky Treats & Snacks:

MEAL PLANNER

WEEK _____

Day	Breakfast	Lunch	Dinner	Dessert
M				
T				
W				
T				
F				
S				
S				

Cheeky Treats & Snacks:

MEAL PLANNER

WEEK _____

Day	Breakfast	Lunch	Dinner	Dessert
M				
T				
W				
T				
F				
S				
S				

Cheeky Treats & Snacks:

MEAL PLANNER

WEEK _____

Day	Breakfast	Lunch	Dinner	Dessert
M				
T				
W				
T				
F				
S				
S				

Cheeky Treats & Snacks:

MEAL PLANNER

WEEK _____

Day	Breakfast	Lunch	Dinner	Dessert
M				
T				
W				
T				
F				
S				
S				

Cheeky Treats & Snacks:

CALORIE JOURNAL

START DATE:

	MON	TUE	WED	THU	FRI	SAT	SUN
BREAKFAST							
LUNCH							
DINNER							
SNACKS							
WATER							
	Total Calories:	Total Calories:	Total Calories:	Total Calories:	Total Calories:	Total Calories:	Total Calories:

CALORIE JOURNAL

START DATE: _____

	MON	TUE	WED	THU	FRI	SAT	SUN
BREAKFAST							
LUNCH							
DINNER							
SNACKS							
WATER							
	Total Calories:	Total Calories:	Total Calories:	Total Calories:	Total Calories:	Total Calories:	Total Calories:

CALORIE JOURNAL

START DATE:

	MON	TUE	WED	THU	FRI	SAT	SUN
BREAKFAST							
LUNCH							
DINNER							
SNACKS							
WATER							
	Total Calories:	Total Calories:	Total Calories:	Total Calories:	Total Calories:	Total Calories:	Total Calories:

CALORIE JOURNAL

START DATE:

	MON	TUE	WED	THU	FRI	SAT	SUN
BREAKFAST							
LUNCH							
DINNER							
SNACKS							
WATER							
	Total Calories:	Total Calories:	Total Calories:	Total Calories:	Total Calories:	Total Calories:	Total Calories:

CALORIE JOURNAL

START DATE:

	MON	TUE	WED	THU	FRI	SAT	SUN
BREAKFAST							
LUNCH							
DINNER							
SNACKS							
WATER							
	Total Calories:	Total Calories:	Total Calories:	Total Calories:	Total Calories:	Total Calories:	Total Calories:

CALORIE JOURNAL

START DATE: _____

	MON	TUE	WED	THU	FRI	SAT	SUN
BREAKFAST							
LUNCH							
DINNER							
SNACKS							
WATER							
	Total Calories:	Total Calories:	Total Calories:	Total Calories:	Total Calories:	Total Calories:	Total Calories:

CALORIE TRACKER

DAILY CALORIE INTAKE

_____

DATE	CAL. COUNT	>	<	=	NOTES

GROCERIES LIST

MONTH: WEEK:

FROZEN
○
○
○
○
○
○
○
○
○
○
○

MEATS / FISH
○
○
○
○
○
○
○
○
○
○
○

PASTA
○
○
○
○
○
○
○
○
○
○
○

FRUITS
○
○
○
○
○
○
○
○
○
○

VEGETABLES
○
○
○
○
○
○
○
○
○
○

DAIRY
○
○
○
○
○
○
○
○
○
○

FOOD LIST

FOOD TO EAT	FOOD TO AVOID
○ _____	○ _____
○ _____	○ _____
○ _____	○ _____
○ _____	○ _____
○ _____	○ _____
○ _____	○ _____
○ _____	○ _____
○ _____	○ _____
○ _____	○ _____
○ _____	○ _____
○ _____	○ _____
○ _____	○ _____
○ _____	○ _____
○ _____	○ _____
○ _____	○ _____
○ _____	○ _____
○ _____	○ _____
○ _____	○ _____
○ _____	○ _____
○ _____	○ _____
○ _____	○ _____
○ _____	○ _____

30 DAYS CHALLENGE

01	02	03	04	05
06	07	08	09	10
11	12	13	14	15
16	17	18	19	20
21	22	23	24	25
26	27	28	29	30

WORKOUT LOG

	Activity	Time	Distance	Sets	Reps	Weight
Monday						
Tuesday						
Wednesday						
Thursday						
Friday						
Saturday						
Sunday						

EXERCISE LOG

DATE:

	EXERCISE	WEIGHT	REPS	SETS	DIST.	TIME
☐						
☐						
☐						
☐						
☐						
☐						
☐						
☐						
☐						
☐						
☐						
☐						
☐						
☐						
☐						
☐						
☐						
☐						
☐						
☐						

STEPS TRACKER

DATE: _____

	1000	2000	3000	4000	5000	6000	7000	8000	9000	10000	11000	12000	13000	14000	15000+
DAY 01															
DAY 02															
DAY 03															
DAY 04															
DAY 05															
DAY 06															
DAY 07															
DAY 08															
DAY 09															
DAY 10															
DAY 11															
DAY 12															
DAY 13															
DAY 14															
DAY 15															
DAY 16															
DAY 17															
DAY 18															
DAY 19															
DAY 20															
DAY 21															
DAY 22															
DAY 23															
DAY 24															
DAY 25															
DAY 26															
DAY 27															
DAY 28															
DAY 29															
DAY 30															
DAY 31															

MONTHLY PROGRESS BAR

HABIT TRACKER

MONTH _____

HABIT:

1	2	3	4	5	6	7
8	9	10	11	12	13	14
15	16	17	18	19	20	21
22	23	24	25	26	27	28
29	30	31				

HABIT:

1	2	3	4	5	6	7
8	9	10	11	12	13	14
15	16	17	18	19	20	21
22	23	24	25	26	27	28
29	30	31				

HABIT:

1	2	3	4	5	6	7
8	9	10	11	12	13	14
15	16	17	18	19	20	21
22	23	24	25	26	27	28
29	30	31				

HABIT:

1	2	3	4	5	6	7
8	9	10	11	12	13	14
15	16	17	18	19	20	21
22	23	24	25	26	27	28
29	30	31				

HABIT:

1	2	3	4	5	6	7
8	9	10	11	12	13	14
15	16	17	18	19	20	21
22	23	24	25	26	27	28

HABIT:

1	2	3	4	5	6	7
8	9	10	11	12	13	14
15	16	17	18	19	20	21
22	23	24	25	26	27	28

WATER TRACKER

MONTH OF

THE WEEK OF	THE WEEK OF	THE WEEK OF	THE WEEK OF

MON

MON

MON

MON

TUE

TUE

TUE

TUE

WED

WED

WED

WED

THU

THU

THU

THU

FRI

FRI

FRI

FRI

SAT

SAT

SAT

SAT

SUN

SUN

SUN

SUN

SLEEP TRACKER

	JAN	FEB	MAR	APR	MAY	JUN	JUL	AUG	SEP	OCT	NOV	DEC
												TOTAL
1	8	9	10	11	**12**	13	14	15	16	17	18	
2	8	9	10	11	**12**	13	14	15	16	17	18	
3	8	9	10	11	**12**	13	14	15	16	17	18	
4	8	9	10	11	**12**	13	14	15	16	17	18	
5	8	9	10	11	**12**	13	14	15	16	17	18	
6	8	9	10	11	**12**	13	14	15	16	17	18	
7	8	9	10	11	**12**	13	14	15	16	17	18	
8	8	9	10	11	**12**	13	14	15	16	17	18	
9	8	9	10	11	**12**	13	14	15	16	17	18	
10	8	9	10	11	**12**	13	14	15	16	17	18	
11	8	9	10	11	**12**	13	14	15	16	17	18	
12	8	9	10	11	**12**	13	14	15	16	17	18	
13	8	9	10	11	**12**	13	14	15	16	17	18	
14	8	9	10	11	**12**	13	14	15	16	17	18	
15	8	9	10	11	**12**	13	14	15	16	17	18	
16	8	9	10	11	**12**	13	14	15	16	17	18	
17	8	9	10	11	**12**	13	14	15	16	17	18	
18	8	9	10	11	**12**	13	14	15	16	17	18	
19	8	9	10	11	**12**	13	14	15	16	17	18	
20	8	9	10	11	**12**	13	14	15	16	17	18	
21	8	9	10	11	**12**	13	14	15	16	17	18	
22	8	9	10	11	**12**	13	14	15	16	17	18	
23	8	9	10	11	**12**	13	14	15	16	17	18	
24	8	9	10	11	**12**	13	14	15	16	17	18	
25	8	9	10	11	**12**	13	14	15	16	17	18	
26	8	9	10	11	**12**	13	14	15	16	17	18	
27	8	9	10	11	**12**	13	14	15	16	17	18	
28	8	9	10	11	**12**	13	14	15	16	17	18	
29	8	9	10	11	**12**	13	14	15	16	17	18	
30	8	9	10	11	**12**	13	14	15	16	17	18	
31	8	9	10	11	**12**	13	14	15	16	17	18	

PERIOD TRACKER

MONTH _____

KEY: ◯ HEAVY   ◯ NORMAL   ◯ LIGHT   ◯ SPOTTING

JANUARY
1 2 3 4 5 6 7 8 9 10 11 12 13 14 15 16 17 18 19 20 21 22 23 24 25 26 27 38 29 30 31

FEBRUARY
1 2 3 4 5 6 7 8 9 10 11 12 13 14 15 16 17 18 19 20 21 22 23 24 25 26 27 38 29 30 31

MARCH
1 2 3 4 5 6 7 8 9 10 11 12 13 14 15 16 17 18 19 20 21 22 23 24 25 26 27 38 29 30 31

APRIL
1 2 3 4 5 6 7 8 9 10 11 12 13 14 15 16 17 18 19 20 21 22 23 24 25 26 27 38 29 30 31

MAY
1 2 3 4 5 6 7 8 9 10 11 12 13 14 15 16 17 18 19 20 21 22 23 24 25 26 27 38 29 30 31

JUNE
1 2 3 4 5 6 7 8 9 10 11 12 13 14 15 16 17 18 19 20 21 22 23 24 25 26 27 38 29 30 31

JULY
1 2 3 4 5 6 7 8 9 10 11 12 13 14 15 16 17 18 19 20 21 22 23 24 25 26 27 38 29 30 31

AUGUST
1 2 3 4 5 6 7 8 9 10 11 12 13 14 15 16 17 18 19 20 21 22 23 24 25 26 27 38 29 30 31

SEPTEMBER
1 2 3 4 5 6 7 8 9 10 11 12 13 14 15 16 17 18 19 20 21 22 23 24 25 26 27 38 29 30 31

OCTOBER
1 2 3 4 5 6 7 8 9 10 11 12 13 14 15 16 17 18 19 20 21 22 23 24 25 26 27 38 29 30 31

NOVEMBER
1 2 3 4 5 6 7 8 9 10 11 12 13 14 15 16 17 18 19 20 21 22 23 24 25 26 27 38 29 30 31

DECEMBER
1 2 3 4 5 6 7 8 9 10 11 12 13 14 15 16 17 18 19 20 21 22 23 24 25 26 27 38 29 30 31

MOOD TRACKER

MONTH _____

1 2 3 4 5 6 7 8 9 10 11 12 13 14 15 16 17 18 19 20 21 22 23 24 25 26 27 28 29 30 31

NEUTRAL

TIRED

STRESSED

GRUMPY

SICK

SAD

RELAXED

HAPPY

ANGRY

NOTES

www.ingramcontent.com/pod-product-compliance
Lightning Source LLC
Chambersburg PA
CBHW070433290526
45791CB00005B/1957